Contents

Introduction 3
    What does the science say? 5
    CBD Oil in Modern History 6
    Market predictions about CBD oil 8
What is CBD Oil? 11
    Is cannabidiol safe? 14
    What is CBD oil exactly? 15
    The CBD Oil Solution 16
        How do you use it? 16
    What is CBD oil used for? 16
    What is CBD oil going for? 18
    How does CBD work? 19
    How do I know if it's really CBD oil in the product? 20
        Should I be wary? 21
        Why are there so many fakes? 21
CBD Oil and Pain 22
CBD Oil for Depression and Anxiety 25
CBD Oil to Quit Smoking 28
CBD Oil and Alzheimer's Disease 30
CBD oil and Parkinson's Disease 32

CBD Oil and Multiple Sclerosis 34
CBD Oil and ALS 35
CBD Oil and Acne 36
CBD Oil and Cancer 38
CBD Oil and Diabetes 41
CBD Oil and Insomnia (Sleep Disorders) 43
CBD oil and Lupus 45
CBD Oil and Crohn's Disease 47
CBD oil and Glaucoma 49
CBD for Huntington's disease 51
CBD Oil and Cardiovascular Diseases 52
CBD Oil and Muscle Spasms 54
CBD Oil and PTSD 55
CBD Oil and Obesity 57
CBD Oil for Asthma 60
CBD Oil for Bipolar Disease 61
CBD Oil for Leukemia 62
CBD Facts You Need To Know 63
   CBD...is it legal? Is it legitimate? Is it safe to consume? 63
CONCLUSION 78
   TAKE AWAY 78

Introduction

Cannabidiol (CBD) is an abundant, non psychoactive, plant derived cannabinoid (phytocannabinoid) whose stereochemistry was first described in 1963 by Mechoulam and colleagues . Isolation of the chemical structure of CBD revealed it to be a classical cannabinoid closely related to cannabinol and tetrahydrocannabinol (THC). A recent review of the safety and side effects of CBD concluded that CBD appears to be well tolerated at high doses and with chronic use in humans, and thus has the potential to be taken safely into the clinic. Indeed, CBD is one of the active ingredients of the currently licensed medication.

CBD oil is the in-thing right now.

It's touted as a natural remedy with a wide range of therapeutic, health and wellness benefits. Thanks to its antipsychotic tendencies, it is also used widely for recreational purposes.Like any cannabis-related product, there's a lot of debate around CBD oil, but that hasn't stopped it from burgeoning to become a $270 million market. And with the Farm Bill 2018 already in force, the best of CBD is yet to come.

Controversial as it might be, the CBD popularity wave has gained increased traction across the country and beyond.

Tons of CBD oil products have found their way into the mainstream market, including CBD vaping cartridges, lip balms, tinctures, and even cosmetics. The pet industry just recently entered the fray, and promises to become one of the biggest consumers of CBD products. Although extensive research has not been done on the subject matter, some of the recent scientific studies seem to suggest that CBD oil has huge potential in treating or managing an array of chronic ailments, such as epilepsy, depression, migraines, cancer, anxiety, and stress.

But, what is CBD oil? Where does it come from? Is it legal to sell market or use it? Is it safe to use it, and how do you use it?

What's its market and future look like? This ultimate guide is dedicated to all things you need to know about CBD oil in 2019, whether you're a consumer, cannabis farmer, prospective investor, dispenser or anyone in between.

What does the science say?

Not much, as far as humans are concerned at least not yet. The vast majority of studies have been on animals, as of yet, and there are few high-quality studies on humans. Even the oil's effect on pain something that CBD oil is popularly used for isn't proven. "The studies available are small or not well designed," says Dr. Devinsky. "There's a lot of religion out there, but not a lot of data."

Dr. Devinsky's research, which was recently published in The New England Journal of Medicine, is beginning to provide that much-needed data in the field of epilepsy research. In a landmark multinational randomized double-blind study for a treatment-resistant form of the condition, subjects taking an oral solution of 20 mg CBD per kilogram of body weight for 14 weeks, along with standard treatment, experienced a 42 percent reduction in drop seizures (the muscles go limp). Those taking a 10 mg CBD per kilogram of body weight saw a 37 percent decrease; patients who got a placebo saw a 17.2 percent decrease. The mechanism hasn't quite been worked out yet, Dr. Devinsky says, though there's some evidence that a receptor known as GPR55 may be critical for the anti-seizure effect.

CBD Oil in Modern History

Hemp was so important to 16th century England that King Henry VIII made it mandatory in 1533 for every farmer to cultivate it. During this period, several physicians including Garcia de Orta started studying the use of hemp extract as an antibiotic and appetite stimulant.

Hemp made it to North America in the 1600s and was also cultivated extensively. In fact, the colony of Virginia made its cultivation mandatory, followed by Connecticut and Massachusetts.

By the 18th century, the medicinal properties and uses of hemp had been documented in the Edinburgh New Dispensatory and The New England Dispensatory. However, it wasn't until 1839 that surgeon William B. O'Shaughnessy started investigating the therapeutic properties of CBD-rich cannabis.

His extensive experiments looked to determine the effects cannabis extracts had on those ailing from hydrophobia, tetanus, cholera, and rheumatic ailments. He unknowingly made way for the discovery of what's now called cannabinoids.

However, it's Robert S Cahn, a British chemist, who is often credited for discovering the first cannabinoid cannabidiol (CBD), which was isolated a couple of years later by US chemist Roger Adams. Adams' research led way to the discovery of THC.

Unfortunately, the war against cannabis hampered further research. When the Control Substance Act was passed in 1970, cultivation of both hemp and marijuana was banned, making it even hard to research or use CBD extract.

The major comeback of CBD oil and hemp extract is largely due to the legalization of medical marijuana across America. Today, the future of CBD oil is brighter than ever.

Market predictions about CBD oil
The CBD oil market is growing rapidly, and its potential for further growth is huge. And it is not just in the United States that CBD oil is raising heads.

With Uruguay and Canada leading the way for the rest of the world in terms of legalizing recreational marijuana, it's just a matter of time before others follow in their footsteps. In the US, Illinois recently became the 11th state to legalize marijuana for adult use. 33 states and Washington have already made it legal for medical purposes.

Widespread legalization of marijuana will certainly fuel the rapid acceptance of CBD oil and related products.

Currently, the cultivation, production, and use of CBD oil are primarily concentrated in Canada, the US and several countries in Europe. In these regions, CBD oil has an established and integrated supply and industry chain, from the hemp and cannabis growers to downstream processors and dispensaries, including a burgeoning list of online stores.

Thanks to this organized chain, a large variety of finished CBD oil products reach the consumer directly and in record time.

However you look at it, CBD oil is poised to become a huge industry. That's not to say the market is currently small. In 2018, the market size for CBD oil was estimated at $270 million.

Prior to 2015, the CBD oil market was relatively small, with the total market sales thought to be valued at around $202 million. Of this, approximately $90 million came from hemp-derived CBD oil products, while the rest (around $112 million) came from the sale of marijuana-derived CBD oil.

According to Brightfield Group market analysis, the sales of hemp-derived CBD oil products jumped to $170 million, registering slightly lower than double growth. Industry experts anticipate that the CBD market will grow at an incredible CAGR of 39.5 percent to hit $3.86 billion by 2025. And yet another market study claims the industry will be worth 20 billion by 2024. This rapid growth is fueled heavily by increased mainstream acceptance.

There are several other predictions for the market, and all seem to paint CBD oil future in a positive light. According to Karnes, the cannabidiol market will hit the $3-billion mark by 2021, while the Brightfield Group says hemp-CBD market alone with reach $22 billion by 2022.

What is CBD Oil?

CBD oil is a popular botanical concentrate that is derived from the cannabis or hemp plant and can vary greatly in color, quality, and clarity depending on the producer. This natural oil extract contains significant amounts of a non-psychotic compound called cannabidiol.

CBD, which is short for cannabidiol, belongs to a class of chemical compounds called cannabinoids that are found a plenty in Cannabis sativa or marijuana plant. In fact, CBD is the second most common of the 104 known cannabinoids found in the cannabis plant.

CBD Oil is not to be mistaken for the much popular relative THC (Tetrahydrocannabinol), which is the most prevalent and active compound in the marijuana plant.

As a psychoactive cannabinoid, THC is best known for delivering a "high" sensation often associated with marijuana when smoked, vaped or ingested.

However, unlike its well-known cousin Tetrahydrocannabinol, cannabidiol (CBD) doesn't have any psychotic effects. In layman terms, CBD oil doesn't make you feel high or alter your brain chemistry like opioids, weed (marijuana) or other psychoactive medical drugs.

This trait makes CBD oil a much safer, milder and a more appealing option for individuals looking for relief from stress, pain, and much more, creating a massive market opportunity for CBD farmers, businesses, researchers and investors alike.

That being said, it's worth mentioning right out of the gate that the terms hemp oil and CBD oil do not refer to the same thing, although the two are often used interchangeably.

Hemp oil is typically extracted by crushing and processing hemp (or industrial hemp) seeds. It comprises no CBD or any other cannabinoid for that matter and is generally used as a dietary supplement or for everyday cooking.

On the other hand, CBD oil is extracted from the flower cluster of either marijuana or hemp plant, depending on the processor. It can also be produced from other parts of the plant.

The cannabidiol oil is often extracted by diluting crushed hemp/cannabis sativa material in a carrier oil like hemp seed oil, jojoba oil, flaxseed oil or coconut oil. More specifically, this oil extract contains lots of cannabidiol, terpenes, and traces of other cannabinoids.

Many states have made CBD oil legal for personal, medical and recreational use.

As such, it's gaining popularity in the health & fitness space, with a number of scientific studies saying it might actually help heal or treat many ailments such as anxiety, depression and chronic pains.

Even still, there's some grey area when it comes to its efficacy, side effects and health potential.

Is cannabidiol safe?
Side effects of CBD include nausea, fatigue and irritability. CBD can increase the level in your blood of the blood thinner coumadin, and it can raise levels of certain other medications in your blood by the exact same mechanism that grapefruit juice does. A significant safety concern with CBD is that it is primarily marketed and sold as a supplement, not

a medication. Currently, the FDA does not regulate the safety and purity of dietary supplements. So you cannot know for sure that the product you buy has active ingredients at the dose listed on the label. In addition, the product may contain other (unknown) elements. We also don't know the most effective therapeutic dose of CBD for any particular medical condition.

What is CBD oil exactly?
CBD or cannabidiol is a type of cannabinoid, a family of molecules typically associated with marijuana, but in fact, also found in other plants and even humans (in us, they're called endocannabinoids). There are hundreds of different cannabinoids in marijuana. The best known is tetrahydrocannabinol, or THC, a chemical in marijuana that targets and binds to certain receptors in the brain to give you a high. CBD is non-psychoactive and non-addictive, and it seems to bind to multiple target sites,

thereby affecting a range of systems throughout the body.

The CBD Oil Solution

How do you use it?

Extracts of CBD either from marijuana or hemp (a cannabis variant that is essentially free of THC) are sold as oil or in tinctures. You can also get CBD via a transdermal patch, capsule, sublingual spray, gel, cream, or vapor. Some contain pure CBD extract (or so they say); others particularly if you're in a state where recreational marijuana is not legal will contain hemp extract, which includes CBD as part of its makeup. As of this reporting, recreational marijuana is legal in nine U.S. states and medical marijuana in 29. Don't miss these 50 weird things that are banned in the United States.

What is CBD oil used for?

Healthy folks vaguely looking to add a little spring in their step (via better sleep, reducing anxiety, or easing muscle soreness) drizzle a little oil into their smoothie or latte. They might also spot-treat with a dab of oil in problematic areas. In the past several years, published papers have suggested that the compound can help with a spectrum of medical conditions, including anxiety, Alzheimer's disease, addiction, arthritis, inflammatory bowel disease, fractures, migraines, psoriasis, and pain. In an animal study, purified extracts of CBD and THC appeared to slow the growth of a type of brain tumor.

"Scientists have been studying other constituents in the marijuana plant beside THC, and there has been an emerging interest in the medical community for a while," says Ryan McLaughlin, PhD, assistant professor of integrative physiology and neuroscience at Washington State University in Pullman.

What is CBD oil going for?

It's not cheap. A vial containing 500 mg of hemp extract from Mary's Nutritionals, for instance, costs $110. CBD extract on its own or as part of a hemp extract, or even with a little THC, if you live in marijuana legal state can be found in a variety of edibles, too, including chocolate bars, honey, and bitters.

"Some products are of little clinical value," says Joanne Miller, a certified nutritionist at Swanson Health Center in Costa Mesa, CA. "But some can be a total game changer in people's lives. There are many, many applications."

Miller, whose clients include patients referred by physicians, uses CBD in a variety of delivery modalities that she has found effective. "Patches can be worn for pain or anxiety management. Capsules or concentrated drops can be taken orally for pain, inflammation, sleep, and anxiety. Balms and creams can be used on the hands and feet to manage arthritic pain.

Vaping is another delivery method," she says.

Her clients require therapeutic doses (generally speaking, 5 to 10 mg per dose), so she recommends brands that have shown results for her clients. Currently, she uses Mary's Medicinals (available in marijuana-legal states) and Thorne.

How does CBD work?
No one's really sure: "It's astonishing that there's still no real consensus on how CBD works," says McLaughlin. "One thing we do know is that it doesn't work through the same receptors as THC, and, in fact, seems to have the opposite effect." THC mainly binds to a certain type of receptor (known as CB1) in the brain. But with CBD, he says, "There seems to be a lot of complex targets" which means CBD may affect multiple pathways throughout the body.

From anecdotal evidence in humans and from animal studies, CBD appears to affect the way we experience pain, inflammation, and anxiety. "Scientists have identified a number of receptors in the nervous system where CBD acts," says Orrin Devinsky, MD, professor of neurology, neurosurgery, and psychiatry at NYU Langone. "It's established that CBD has anti-inflammatory properties and can increase activity at some serotonin [the feel-good neurotransmitter] receptors."

How do I know if it's really CBD oil in the product?
Unfortunately, you don't. Even though more than half of all U.S. states now allow marijuana for medicinal purposes and nine of those, plus Washington DC, allow it for recreational use the Drug Enforcement Agency still views CBD as a banned substance and therefore doesn't regulate it (since, in the eyes of the law, CBD shouldn't be on the market). "I can start a company, put oil in a jar and sell it as CBD oil," says McLaughlin and no one

has to vouch that what's in there is for real. You have only the manufacturers' word for it.

Should I be wary?
Yes: CBD extracts can't always be trusted. A 2017 JAMA paper reported that almost 70 percent of all CBD products sold online do not contain the amount of CBD stated on the label. Of the 84 products bought from 31 different companies, 42 percent contained a higher concentration of CBD oil than the label claimed, and 26 percent of the products contained less than the label claimed. The remainders of products contained the labeled amount give or take 10 percent.

Why are there so many fakes?
"There's no oversight," says Marcel Bonn-Miller, PhD, adjunct assistant professor of Psychology in Psychiatry at the University of Pennsylvania and author of the JAMA article. Beyond the label, he adds,

"There's no consistency. You know that every Hershey's bar you buy and every Coke you buy will be exactly the same. But that's not the case with the majority of CBD products. It's not unexpected to see variability within a given brand." This means that you may notice improvements the first time you buy and try a particular product, but none the next.

"There's no way to know what you're getting unless you bring the product yourself to a reputable lab and get it analyzed," says Bonn-Miller.

CBD Oil and Pain
Use of CBD-rich cannabis to alleviate or manage pain is something that goes way back. In fact, there's evidence that CBD-rich marijuana has been used to relieve pain dating as far back as 2900 BC.

But how does CBD oil help with pain? As mentioned above, the pain-relieving effects of CBD oil can be explained by its ability to interact with cannabinoid receptors in your body.

Our body has a highly specialized system known as the endocannabinoid system (ECS) that is responsible for several different functions, including appetite, sleep, immune response, and pain. By binding with CB2 receptors, CBD helps influence this system and encourage the production of more serotonin and melatonin (more on this below).

As explained earlier, serotonin is a remarkable neurotransmitter. It's a class of what is called 'happy-feel" hormones, alongside endorphins and dopamine. It has almost the same effects on your brain as opioids.

Serotonin helps soothe pain centers in the brain and central nervous system. That's exactly why you tend to feel relaxed, calm and feel a rush of a pain-relieving wave when you take CBD.

There are also several studies that have shown that CBD oil is effective when it comes to dealing with chronic pain, especially those associated with cancers, spinal cord injuries, migraines, arthritis, muscle pain, MS pain and so forth.

In a 2011 study, researchers discovered that CBD helps reduce inflammatory pain (or arthritis pain, to be precise) in lab rats. They further found that it does so by influencing the way pain receptors respond to underlying cause/stimuli.

An extensive review conducted in 2014 concluded that CBD might be a viable treatment option for osteoarthritis (OA) pain.

As there is no existing traditional medication to help control or manage the progression and pain associated with OA, CBD oil may come in especially useful. Another study carried out a couple of years later confirmed that CBD has the potential of relieving inflammation and pain linked to arthritis when applied topically.

If that is not clear enough, there's another 2017 study on rats which revealed that CBD oil may be much safer and more effective at treating osteoarthritis joint pain than other available treatment options.

Besides animal studies, a number of studies on human subjects have shown that a combo of THC and CBD is a useful treatment for pain associated with sciatic nerve issues, rheumatoid arthritis, and multiple sclerosis.

NIH (National Institute of Health) has also funded or co-sponsored several preclinical studies and trials to help understand the role of CBD-rich cannabis in managing or relieving pain and other symptoms related to back pain, chronic pain, arthritis, etc.

CBD Oil for Depression and Anxiety

In 2015 alone, it is estimated that over 16 million American adults experienced major depressive episodes. Anxiety is another rampant mental health problem in America, affecting more than 18.1 percent of the entire population of the country.

Additionally, The World Health Organization says anxiety disorders are ranked 6th, while depression is the single biggest cause of disability across the globe.

To add insult to injury, pharma meds used to treat depression and anxiety are usually riddled with side effects, including insomnia, aggression, drowsiness, nausea, reduced sex drive, and headaches that won't quit.

Some opioid treatment options also lead to serious substance abuse and addiction. That's why more and more people are turning to CBD products.

CBD's ability to increase the levels of serotonin in the body can help reduce symptoms of depression and keep anxiety at bay. And there are several scientific studies that seem to concur.

For example, in a 2014 study, de Mello Schier AR and his team at the Federal University of Rio de Janeiro found that CBD has significant anxiolytic (anti-anxiety) and antidepressant-like properties.

Earlier, in a 2011 study, his counterparts from the Department of Neurosciences and Behavior, Division of Psychiatry, University of São Paulo had used both human and animals models to demonstrate cannabidiol oil's effectiveness in treating social anxiety disorder.

In this comprehensive study, 24 individuals with social anxiety disorder were given treatment solution containing around 600mg of cannabidiol before going to give a public speech. Some of them didn't receive CBD.

Those who took CBD were less anxious and experienced much fewer speech issues or cognitive impairment when giving their speeches than those who didn't.

In a 2016 study, Scott Shannon and his fellow researchers at the University of Colorado School of Medicine in Fort Collins demonstrated that CBD oil can be safely and effectively used to treat anxiety and sleep disorders in children with PTSD.

Bottom line: CBD oil has been found through several studies to help reduce depression and anxiety disorders in both animals and humans. Its antidepressant and anti-anxiety qualities are linked to the cannabinoids' ability to influence receptors for serotonin, a hormone that regulates social behavior, mood and one's general state of happiness.

CBD Oil to Quit Smoking

Tobacco smoking can cause insurmountable damage to the smoker's health and well-being. It's a risk factor for heart disease, bronchitis, glaucoma, infertility, sexual dysfunction, diabetes, hypertension, and several cancers.

The good news is that 68 percent of smokers in the US want to quite. But smoking cessation is not an easy walk in the park. Of course, the last thing you want is to quit cold turkey.

CBD oil has shown great potential to lessen the level of reward smoker's brain gets from smoking tobacco, and therefore loosening their dependency on them. It acts like a nicotine patch but without all the side effects and withdrawal symptoms.

A 2013 study found that CBD treatment can indeed reduce one's dependence on nicotine or tobacco smoking. In this study, 12 smokers were issued with inhalers infused with CBD oil, while the other 12 participants were given non-CBD inhalers.

Those who used CBD-rich inhalers reduced the number of cigarettes smoked per day by an average of 40 percent. There was no difference in those that didn't use CBD.

In another comprehensive 2015 study, researchers discovered that CBD has multi-prong benefits that can help smokers quit smoking, including reducing social anxiety disorders, withdrawal syndrome, and other metrics related to addiction.

Moreso, CBD helps with depression and relaxes the nerves, which is always a big plus for anyone attempting to cease smoking.

CBD Oil and Alzheimer's Disease
Alzheimer's disease is a neurodegenerative disorder that's characterized by severe memory loss and damage to other brain functions. It's common among seniors aged 65+ and is the leading cause of dementia (responsible for 60-80 percent).There is no known cure for Alzheimer's disease.

The good news is that CBD oil has shown a great deal of potential to benefit Alzheimer's sufferers. According to CBD Kyro, long-term use of CBD oil is much tolerable and can help treat underlying symptoms like aggression and agitation, as well as root causes.

In one study carried out in 2014, mice genetically predisposed to the disease received CBD treatment every day for 8 months. The researchers were excited to discover that CBD helped the mice by reducing the effects of Alzheimer's disease. Their ability to recognize faces increased, social withdrawals reduced and overall cognitive deficits decreased.

Several other test-tube and animal model studies have proved that CBD oil has great potential to reduce inflammation and thus help prevent cognitive degeneration often linked to Alzheimer's disease.

The scientists believe that CBD's action on receptors in the brain and immune system is responsible for reducing inflammation in the nerves, lowering cholesterol levels, and increased retention of important nutrients.

CBD oil and Parkinson's Disease

Parkinson's Disease (PD) is a serious neurological disorder that worsens progressively with time and age. It affects primarily the nervous system, adversely impacting mobility, speech and motor skills.

Like Alzheimer's Disease, there's no cure for PD, but there's a growing list of medications and options that can be used to manage the symptoms and improve quality of life. CBD oil has joined that list.

Unlike most meds meant for PD management, however, CBD oil doesn't come with serious side effects like ankle swelling, insomnia, liver damage, urinary problems, constipation, diarrhea, skin blotching, and nausea.

CBD has also been studied extensively for its potential benefits in treating PD.

For instance, two 2014 studies revealed that long-term and consistent treatment with CBD oil enhanced sleep quality and spruced up the quality of life for individuals living with Parkinson's Disease.

In another 2014 study, 22 people with Parkinson's Disease who received CBD-rich cannabis saw significant improvement in pain, tremors, sleep, and mobility. These impressive benefits were noticed within just 30 minutes of using cannabis.

In yet another groundbreaking study published in 2010, scientists discovered that CBD and other cannabinoids can help with inflammation, which is often associated with PD.

As a non-psychoactive cannabinoid, CBD might help in several ways to manage or reduce PD symptoms. Of course, the research into the potential benefits of CBD oil for Parkinson's Disease is ongoing.

CBD Oil and Multiple Sclerosis

Multiple sclerosis (MS) is a progressive neurodegenerative disease that's depicted by the damage of nerve cells in the spinal cord and the brain.

Its symptoms may include speech impairment, blurred vision, muscular miscoordination, tremors, jerking, weakness, and persistent fatigue and numbness, all of which can lead to a serious disability.

There are several FDA-approved therapies available to mitigate symptoms of MS, but most of them come with some side effects. Good thing, a number of recent studies on the use of CBD have shown promising outcomes.

For example, 5 extensive reviews discussed at the Consortium of MS Centers in Tennessee lead to the conclusion that there's enough evidence CBD can be a viable treatment option for involuntary muscle contraction, tremors, and pain associated with MS.

Another study published in 2014 found that Sativex, a CBD-rich oral spray is a not only effective but also a safe way to ameliorate muscle spasticity in multiple sclerosis patients. Of the 276 participants, 75 percent experienced a reduction in muscle spasticity after using Sativex. What's more, their spasms had developed resistance to conventional drugs.

A 2012 study also found that Nabiximols containing CBD-rich cannabis can help treat spasticity, urinary, and pain linked to MS.

CBD Oil and ALS
Amyotrophic Lateral Sclerosis (Lou Gehrig's disease), or ALS for short, is a debilitating neurological condition that affects the spinal cord and motor neurons. It causes progressive weakness of one's muscle system.

About 30,000 Americans have ALS, with global sufferers numbering around 450,000. Currently, there's no effective treatment of ALS, with the focus of research now on CBD and other cannabinoids like THC.

In a study published in 2009, Chandrasekaran Raman and his team at the Forbes Norris MDA/ALS Research discovered that use of CBD oil helped delay the progression of ALS in mice. Specifically, muscle weakening reduced by half when the mice were treated with cannabidiol.

This hinges on one study by a team from the Neurological Clinics, Department of Neurosciences at the University of Rome, which found the link between ALS and problems in the endocannabinoid system (ECS).

CBD Oil and Acne
Affecting over 9 percent of Americans, acne is a pretty common skin blemish that can be unsightly and uncomfortable

to many. It is caused by inflammation in the skin cells and other parts of the body.

Common risk factors and causes include over secretion of sebum, inflammation, bacterial infection and genetics. CBD oil has shown promising results when it comes to treating and managing acne.

In an extensive 2014 study published in the Journal of Clinical Investigation, Attila Oláh and his team showed that CBD oil can help prevent over-activity in glands responsible for the production of sebum. This way, the oil prevents acne flare-ups, while keeping the skin sufficiently moist.

Another study published in same year found that CBD helps prevent acne-activating agents (such as cytokines), induced anti-inflammatory reactions, and inhibited sebaceous glands from producing too much sebum.

Scientists believe that CBD is a safe and effective acne treatment because of its ability to not only dial down sebum secretion, but also its anti-inflammatory qualities. Of course, users are recommended to seek advice from their doctors or dermatologists before using CBD regimens.

CBD Oil and Cancer

It is no big secret that cancer is a growing tumor in the US. According Center for Disease Control, 1.6 million Americans are diagnosed with some form of cancer, and 600,000 succumb to the disease every year.

Cancer treatments and therapies like chemotherapy have devastating side effects and they aren't exactly effective. Which begs the question: is CBD oil the answer?

This 2012 study says CBD can help fight cancer directly. The study seems to conclude that CBD has anti progressive, anti-migratory, anti-metastatic and anti-invasive properties against cancer.

While that might be refutable, most research studies admit that, at a minimum, CBD helps with managing some cancer-related symptoms.

For example, one study published in 2010 investigated the effects of CBD-rich cannabis on 177 cancer patients. The vast majority of these people couldn't get pain relief from conventional medication.

Those who received CBD-rich treatment experienced a notable decrease in cancer-related pain, nausea and sleep problems. In fact, these benefits were greater in CBD recipients than those who were treated with an extract containing only THC.

Several test-tube studies and those done on animal subjects have also revealed that CBD might have anti-cancer qualities after all. For instance, a 2011 research study demonstrated that high CBD extract can trigger the death of human breast cancer cells.

In another study done in 2007, scientists found out that CBD can reduce the spreading and progression of aggressive breast cancer cells in mice, by a huge margin. While these studies are indeed groundbreaking, scientists are yet to replicate these results in the human body.

Some animal and human studies have also shown that CBD can help decrease chemotherapy side effects like vomiting and nausea.

In a study published in the British Journal of Clinical Pharmacology, 16 cancer patients going through chemo used an oral spray ladened with CBD-rich cannabis an average of 4.8 times per day. 71.4 percent of patients who usedCBD spray said they experienced a reduction in vomiting and nausea.

Bottom line: An array of animal, test-tube and human studies has shown that CBD has potential anti-cancer properties.

While it can help reduce symptoms and conditions associated to cancer and cancer treatment, further research is required to review CBD's safety and effectiveness.

CBD Oil and Diabetes

Gestational, type 1 and type 2 diabetes are a growing concern for Americans and healthcare providers. According to the CDC, over 84 million American adults are diabetic or pre-diabetic, but only 10 percent are aware that they have it.

If you do the math, you'll find out that more than one-third of Americans will have to face diabetes at some point. In fact, this chronic condition is the seventh most lethal disease when it comes to killing Americans.

Of all the forms of diabetes, type 2 is responsible for between 90 and 95 percent of all diagnosed cases – most of the rest goes to type 1 diabetes.

More and more people are opting for CBD oil as a treatment option for their condition. Some use it to manage their precarious condition. And there's a growing batch of studies that show that CBD is an effective choice for treating type 2 diabetes.

One interesting study published in 2013 in the American Journal of Medicine drew several conclusion about CBD use for diabetes treatment. It concluded that CBD users have high levels of HDL (the good cholesterol) despite eating a regular diet. More importantly, the study confirmed that CBD might help regulate blood sugar, which is crucial to managing type 2 diabetes.

More recent research conducted in 2016 discovered that mice predisposed to diabetes developed type 1 diabetes much later than expected, showed marginally reduced signs oxidation (inflammation) and had significantly increased the production of insulin in the pancreas when they were treated with CBD oil.

In an earlier study, researchers found that CBD treatment can prevent 56 percent of diabetic mice from developing diabetes. As if that wasn't incredible enough, the study uncovered that CBD also helped significantly reduce inflammation in diabetic mice.

Bottom line: While these studies have shown that CBD might be an effective treatment route for diabetes, more research is needed to be carried out in humans.

CBD Oil and Insomnia (Sleep Disorders)

Getting at least 7 hours of restful sleep is important for your health and well-being. Unfortunately, more Americans are short sleepers than ever before.

Lack of enough sleep or suffering from insomnia can lead to a devastating impact on your mental, physical and emotional well-being. In fact, several studies have shown that people who suffer from insomnia tend to be obese, are physically inactive and often turn to smoke.

Insomnia can affect your immune system, can lead to depression, and can become a risk factor for heart disease, diabetes, and other chronic conditions.

CBD oil and can help, and several animals, human and in-vitro studies agree. CBD oil action on serotonin in the brain helps reduce depression, anxiety, chronic pain, inflammation, seizures, and digestion problem, all of which are known causes of insomnia.

Serotonin is a powerful hormone that returns your parasympathetic centers in your brain to its relaxed and calm state. This way, you can go to nod land without any trouble.

CBD oil also helps encourage the production of melatonin, a well-known hormone that aids sleep. It helps you not only fall asleep faster but also sleep longer and get a restful night.

In a 2013 study, researchers treated mice with CBD and monitored their sleep factors. They found out that mice thatwere treated with CBD experienced increased sleep latency when exposed to light. It also increases total sleep duration.

Another study published in 2014 looked to establish if cannabidiol could help treat obstructive sleep apnea, which affects close to 100 million people worldwide. The findings show that CBD induced serotonin production, which help reduce sleep apnea in mice.

CBD oil and Lupus

Lupus is the disease of the immune system that's characterized by pain, swelling, inflammation, joint issues, rash, fever, and fatigue. According to the Lupus Foundation of America, more than 1.5 million people in the US have lupus, with 90 percent being women.

Current treatment options for lupus are unreliable and most of them lead to opioid addiction. A growing list of research initiatives seems to suggest that CBD oil can be an effective and safe treatment for inflammation and pain related to lupus.

There are also several studies and anecdotal evidence that CBD oil helps manage lupus by acting on T-cells. For example, in a study published in 2018 in the Cellular Immunology, scientists found that CBD changes the way T-cells function when given to someone with a spinal cord injury.

Lupus is often associated with chronic pain from nerve damage, and several studies show that cannabidiol oil can help relieve a wide range of pains. This type of pain is often linked to rheumatoid arthritis,

HIV, migraines, spinal cord injury, and much more.

CBD Oil and Crohn's Disease

Crohn's disease is a painful type of IBS (irritable bowel syndrome) that affects the gastrointestinal tract, particularly the small intestine. It's not only extremely painful but can also be quite disabling.

It is typically symptomized by bleeding from the rectum, diarrhea, abdominal cramps, persistent constipation, and frequent need to move bowels. If not treated early, it can lead to extreme weight loss, abnormal menstruation cycle, fatigue, grave loss of appetite and excessive sweating at night.

Crohn's& Colitis Foundation (CCF), more than 780,000 people in the US have Crohn'sdiseaese. Risk factors include environmental, genetics, stress and poor diet. It is quite common in young adults and adolescents.

Immune modifiers, antibiotics, and sometimes steroids are often prescribed to help fend off inflammation and manage the condition. CBD oil is touted as the perfect candidate for alleviating pain, stress and other symptoms and perceived causatives of Crohn's disease.

In a first of its kind study that was presented at the United European Gastroenterology conference, scientists found that CBD-rich cannabis can help reduce clinical remission for Crohn's Disease sufferers by 50 percent after 8 weeks of use.

Moreover, 65 percent of participants said CBD helped them reduce IBD symptoms as well as improve their quality of life. As such, researchers have demonstrated that CBD oil can deliver measurable results and improvements in controlling Crohn's disease symptoms.

According to lead researcher, Dr. TimnaNaftali, CBD oil can play a key role in slowing the movement of food in the gut, increasing appetite, reducing pain, preventing diarrhea, and reducing intestinal secretion.

While the study has not been officially published, the findings are remarkable. It will become the base study for further research from now henceforth.

CBD oil and Glaucoma

Glaucoma is one of the leading eye conditions, affecting more than 3 million people in the US.

Glaucoma is the 2nd leading cause of lost eyesight across the world, only trailing cataract. The most unfortunate part is that about half of people with glaucoma don't know that they have it.

It so happens that CBD oil can help you prevent glaucoma from stealing your eyesight. And most studies that have been carried out over the years are in agreement with this statement.

For instance, milestone research conducted in 1971 investigated the effect of CBD on eye pressure in young people. Increased eye pressure is often one of the most apparent symptoms of glaucoma which have adverse damage to the optic nerve, causing the subject to lose eyesight with time.

According to the study, scientists found out subjects who used CBD experienced a decrease in eye pressure of around 30 percent. As exciting as that may seem, that's just but the tip of the iceberg of how CBD can help tackle glaucoma.

In another study published in 1978, it was found that the use of CBD-rich cannabis can cause significant reduction in intraocular (optic nerve) pressure both in human subjects and dogs with glaucoma.

In another comprehensive study reviewing CBD and glaucoma studies conducted between 1997 and 2008, the authors concluded that cannabidiol helps reduce not only eye pressure but also toxicity in the retina of an eye. Both conditions can worse glaucoma if they are not tamed.

CBD for Huntington's disease

Huntington's disease, or simply HD, is a neurodegenerative genetic disorder that causes the breakdown of the brain's nerve cells. It is described as an anomaly in eye movements, slow eyesight, rigid muscles, writhing movements, and jerking motions.

If not controlled early enough, HD will render the person unable to speak, walk or reason with time. Only 1 percent of Americans are at the risk of developing Huntington's disease. CBD oil is chock-full of health and medical benefits that can prove useful in the fight against HD.

A 2011 study showed that the use of CBD can help reduce the progression of HD. And results from this clinical trial show positive outcomes. The patients who used CBD extract experienced less muscle spasticity; eye movements were sharper and saw lower jerking movements.

CBD Oil and Cardiovascular Diseases
Heart disease is one the leading causes of death in America. Every 40 seconds someone has a stroke or heart attack in the US. And with increase of lifestyle conditions, cardiovascular diseases will keep US healthcare industry busy for several years to come.

The good news is that myriads of research and groundbreaking studies have linked CBD oil with numerous health benefits for your ticker, blood flow and circulation system. Perhaps the most crucial benefit is its ability to regulate blood sugar and pressure.

A 2014 high blood pressure review study established the link between hypertension and issues with metabolism, heart attack and stroke. Good thing, there is a multitude of studies that seem to indicate that CBD oil may be a safe, natural and effective solution for hypertension (high blood pressure).

Take this study that was published in 2017, for instance. 10 healthy male participants were given either a placebo or 600mg of CBD. The researchers discovered that CBD helps reduce resting (what's called basal) blood pressure. Scientists concluded that the anti-anxiety and anti-stress properties of cannabidiol were responsible for its ability to bring down blood pressure.

Furthermore, many test-tube and animal subject studies have show that CBD can indeed help not only prevent death of cardiovascular cells but also reduce inflammation which is often associated with heart disease.

For example, in one 2010 study, researchers found that using CBD to treat diabetic mice with cardiovascular disease help reduce oxidative stress (which is linked to inflammation) and prevent heart failure. They believe that the powerful antioxidant and anti-stress properties lead to its ability to prevent heart damage.

CBD Oil and Muscle Spasms

Related to Multiple Sclerosis (MS), CBD can also help with muscle spasms.

Traditionally, muscles relaxants like Valium are used as quick fixes for muscle tension, soreness, pain, and spasm. But remember most of these muscle medications are either riddled with side effects, ineffective or lead to substance abuse and addiction.

There are numerous research and studies that depict CBD as a great muscle relaxant.

For instance, a study published in Neurotherapeutics in 2015 noticed that CBD has significant potential as a treatment option for muscle spasticity, tension, rigidity and other conditions that result from poor workouts, overwork or chronic stress.

In another 2015 study, 47 individuals with muscle spasm as a result of Multiple Sclerosis experienced a significant reduction in muscle rigidity, increased walking and reduced pain when treated with Sativex, an oral treatment that is laced with CBD. It also led to great improvement in sleep quality and less pain during movement.

Bottom line: Muscle spasm can be not only painful but can also impact on your quality of life. CBD-rich cannabis extract has been found to be effective when it comes to decreasing this pain linked to muscles spasms, rheumatoid arthritis, and MS.

CBD Oil and PTSD

It is estimated that 3.6 percent of Americans have experienced Post Traumatic Stress Disorder (PTSD).

Women are at a greater risk of PTSD causes.

Going through the motions of PTSD can be quite unsettling. That's why more and more war veterans and other PTSD sufferers are turning to cannabinoids like CBD for relief and to get by.

Some studies have found that CBD may be safe and effective in providing relief from post-traumatic stress and managing PTSD in general.

By acting on or influencing CB2 receptors and inducing production of serotonin, CBD plays a key role in helping people suffering from PTSD by preventing them from retrieving their nightmares and traumatic memories.

CBD also helps PTSD sufferers stay on top of their mental health by reducing anxiety, stress, depression and other factors that are essential for emotional well-being. This is especially true for combat veterans who want to forget painful memories.

In one study carried out by the researchers at NYU Langone Medical Center, it was revealed that combat veterans suffering from PTSD have extremely low levels of anandamide, a neurotransmitter that has an high affinity for CB2 receptors. What that means is that these patients can use CBD oil (preferably in conjunction with cannabis) to increase their serotonin and anandamide levels.

Numerous other studies have also demonstrated how CBD treatment helps reduce memory of fear, stress circulation, conditioned fear, and even reversing development of PTSD.

CBD Oil and Obesity

Close to 40 percent of adult Americans are either obese or close to being overweight. This can present a huge lifestyle and health challenges. After all, obesity is a risk factor for type 2 diabetes, stroke, cardiovascular disease, hypertension, and several kinds of cancer.

Obesity is preventable, but beating it isn't always a picnic.

Enter CBD oil, an extract which can help obese people burn unwanted fat, lose weight and keep it off. There are many scientific studies that demonstrate how CBD helps people suffering from obesity lose weight:

Fat conversion: Some studies suggest that CBD helps convert bad (white) fat into favorable (brown) fat that is easy for the body to zap. Moreover, white fat is often associated with increased risk of chronic ailments like diabetes and heart disease.

In a study published in 2016, scientists zeroed in on the possibility that CBD plays a crucial role in how our body deals with fat. They found that CBD does this in two ways: (1) it helps the creation of easily metabolized brown fat cells from white ones, and (2) it revs up metabolism making it burn more fat.

Curbs raging appetite: Most obese people have an uncontrolled appetite which forces them to go an eating spree or binging. CB1's antagonizing effects of CBD help obese people curb their big appetites and therefore cut weight.

In other words, CBD molecules help block off CB1 receptors, which are responsible for increased appetite, from being activated. A 2012 study showed that CBD exposure to rates helped suppress their appetite.

Controlling metabolic disorders: a top-down review published in the Cannabis and Cannabinoid Research journal showcases and analyzes the bulk of existing studies that surround the link between metabolic disorders and CBD.

CBD Oil for Asthma

Asthma is one of the most common chronic conditions of the respiratory system. This lung condition is occurs when the airways in the lungs are inflamed, forcing them to constrict and filled up with phlegm. That's why someone with asthma find it difficult to breath and their lungs usually wheeze during breathing.

Over 25 million people in the US have asthma, as per the National Heart, Lung, and Blood Institute. Most of the asthma sufferers are looking for safer, more natural alternatives to inhalers. And that's where CBD oil comes into the picture.

A burgeoning body of studies and research is focusing on CBD's effects on asthma.

A 2012 study on the effects of CBD on asthma found that it reduces inflammation resulting from allergic reactions, reduces pain associated with asthma, and heal the nerves affected by inflammation.

These findings are in line with a 2011 study that showed that allergen exposure leads to increase in neurotransmitters like anandamide which can be blocked off by CBD.

CBD Oil for Bipolar Disease

5 million individuals in the US (or about 2.8 percent of the population) suffer from bipolar disorders.

These are rare brain or mental health conditions that are typified by extreme mood swings or changes, which include high, manic episodes and low, depressive episodes. These episodes can last for many days or weeks on end.

Mood swings resulting from bipolar disorders can be precarious and extreme. Such a person may experience symptoms of psychosis-like delusions and hallucinations. A growing volume of studies shows that CBD can also help with bipolar disorders.

CBD oil helps improve mood and reduce mental impairment: in a 2016 study, researchers found that bipolar people experienced fewer mental impairments and had a better mood when they used CBD oil. Although most naysayers say cannabinoids can affect memory and thinking, this study seems to show otherwise.

CBD oil promotes a positive outlook: A study published in 2015 showed that CBD use in persons diagnosed with a bipolar condition helped improve not only their mood but also led them to have a more optimistic outlook on life. In other words, they tend to have a better day when they are on treatment with CBD-rich cannabis.

CBD Oil for Leukemia

Leukemia is the cancer of red blood cells or the bone marrow. It progresses aggressively, and eventually reduces your body's ability to fend off infection and intruders. Only 57 percent of people with leukemia survive after 5 years with the disease.

More than 60,000 new cases of leukemia are discovered in the US every year, with around 23,000 succumbing to cancer. Thankfully, researchers are now finding out that CBD oil can improve the chances of survival.

In a study published in 2005, Catherine Lombard and her team at the Department of Microbiology and Immunology, Medical College of Virginia showed that leukemia cells can be targeted using CBD via cannabinoid receptors. This study found that CBD can help reduce activators and progression of the disease.

CBD Facts You Need To Know

CBD...is it legal? Is it legitimate? Is it safe to consume?
1.) CBD is a Main Component of Cannabis

Cannabidiol (CBD) is a primary component of cannabis. It is one of more than 85 compounds unique to the plant and grouped under the umbrella term cannabinoids. CBD and THC are the most prominent cannabinoids found in cannabis, and as such have undergone the heaviest scientific study.

2.) CBD Oil Won't Get You High

CBD does not cause the feeling of being high that is often associated with cannabis. The high is caused by THC. THC binds tightly to the CB1 and CB2 nerve receptors in the brain and throughout the body. CBD does not bind to these receptors and instead causes its therapeutic actions through more indirect means.

Because CBD will not make you feel intoxicated, it is a great option for parents, workers, and anyone else who does not to compromise their mental clarity.

Much health conditions, both severe and not, are treated with pharmaceutical drugs. Unfortunately, many of these drugs have unpleasant or dangerous side effects. In some instances, CBD may offer non-toxic, virtually side-effect free, natural benefits for individuals who want to avoid or reduce the number of pharmaceuticals they are taking.

3.) CBD Oil from Hemp is Legal

CBD products come either from medical cannabis or industrial hemp plants. While still illegal under federal law, cannabis is legal in several states. And because it has a low THC content (>.3%), industrial hemp does not fall under these same regulations. This means that consumers are free to choose CBD as a natural supplement without worrying about any legal repercussions.

4.) The Human Body Produces Cannabinoids, and CBD Oil Helps

Phytocannabinoids are cannabinoids derived from plants. Endocannabinoids are cannabinoids produced naturally in the human body.

One example of an endocannabinoid is anandamide, or 'the bliss molecule.' This molecule activates the CB1 receptor.

Benefits of activating the CB1 receptor include:

Relieving depression

Increasing myelin formation

Lowering intestinal inflammation

Decreasing intestinal permeability (Leaky Gut Syndrome)

Lowering blood pressure

Lowering anxiety

Reducing fear and paranoia

Increasing BDNF levels

Increasing PPARy expression

Reducing GPR55 signaling

Lowering prolactin

An enzyme in the body known as FAAH is responsible for breaking down anandamide. CBD is an inhibitor of FAAH, meaning more anandamide to be available to the CB1 receptors.

Anandamide has been shown to stop the proliferation of breast cancer cells, promote anti-anxiety and antidepressant effects, and increases neurogenesis. Anandamide plays a role in memory and forgetting, creating a potential natural value for individuals with post traumatic stress disorder (PTSD).

5.) CBD Oil Effects Several Neurotransmitter Receptors

CBD is an allosteric modulator at several receptor sites in our bodies.

Allosteric modulators change the shape of specific receptors to alter their ability to interact with neurotransmitters.

CBD is a positive allosteric modulator of the mu and delta opioid receptors. This means it enhances the ability of these receptors to receive endogenous enkephalins which can increase quality of life and naturally reduce pain. Inversely, CBD is a negative allosteric modulator of the CB1 receptor, reducing its ability to bind with THC; this explains why high-CBD cultivars of cannabis mitigate many of the unwanted side effects associated with THC.

At high doses, CBD activates the 5-ht1A receptor. The 5-ht1A receptor helps regulate anxiety, addiction, appetite, sleep, pain perception, nausea, and vomiting. CBDA (the raw form of CBD) shows an even higher affinity for the 5-ht1A receptor than CBD.

CBD also antagonizes GPR55 receptors. GPR55 receptors are widely distributed in the brain (especially the cerebellum) and help to control bone density and blood pressure. When activated, GPR55 promotes cancer cell proliferation. This antagonizing action may help explain the natural value of supplementing with CBD in individuals with cancer, osteoporosis, and high blood pressure.

CBD activates TRPV1 receptors. TRPV1 is involved in regulating pain, body temperature, and inflammation. Other substances targeting TRPV1 receptors include anandamide, AM404 (a metabolite of acetaminophen), capsaicin, and various cannabinoids such as CBN, CBG, CBC, THCV, and CBDV.

Lastly, CBD activates PPAR-gamma receptors. PPAR-gamma receptors are located on the cell's nuclei and play a role in lipid uptake, insulin sensitivity, dopamine release and the degradation of beta-amyloid plaque. This is why CBD has been found to have natural value for individuals with diabetes, schizophrenia, and Alzheimer's disease.

6.) CBD Oil May Help with Clinical Endocannabinoid Deficiency (CECD)

Clinical Endocannabinoid Deficiency is a condition where an individual has a lower amount of endogenous cannabinoids than is considered necessary to promote health and well-being.

Scientists now believe CECD may play a role in the following conditions:

Fibromyalgia

Irritable Bowel Syndrome (IBS)

Migraines

Multiple Sclerosis (MS)

Post-Traumatic Stress Disorder (PTSD)

Neuropathy

Huntington's

Parkinson's

Motion Sickness

Autism

Many of these conditions are treated with a range of medications that carry some heavy side effects. As the research develops, if CECD is found to be the culprit behind these conditions, CBD would help increase endocannabinoids in the body without many of the risks associated with pharmaceuticals.

7.) CBD Oil Has Numerous Natural Benefits

Cannabidiol is one of 85+ cannabinoids found in the cannabis plant, and much of the ongoing research has found it to be a promising potential therapy for many illnesses that medical professionals have previously thought to be untreatable, including:

Pain (neuropathic, chronic, cancer-related, etc.)

Epilepsy

Multiple Sclerosis (MS)

Amyotrophic Lateral Sclerosis (ALS)

Parkinson's

Inflammation

Acne

Dyskinesia

Psoriasis

Broken Bones

Mad Cow Disease

Depression

Bacterial Infections

Diabetes

Rheumatoid Arthritis

Nausea

Anxiety

ADHD

Schizophrenia

Substance Abuse/Withdrawal

Heart Disease

Irritable Bowel Syndrome (IBS)

8.) CBD Is But One Part of the Entourage Effect

The entourage effect describes the phenomenon where the 400+ compounds in cannabis work in concert to have a synergistic effect on the body. In other words, it is the sum of its parts that make cannabis so effective.

For example, 100mg of isolated CBD may be substantially less effective at alleviating symptoms than 100mg of a whole-plant, cannabis extract.

Vitamin C may be a good analogy. Many vitamin C supplements are presented in the form of ascorbic acid. Ascorbic acid is just one of the many compounds that comprise the whole vitamin C. In order to be most effective, vitamin C must also exist alongside rutin, Factor K, Factor J, Factor P, Tyrosinase, and Ascorbigen. In fact, in all of his years of research, the discoverer of Vitamin C and Nobel prize laureate Dr. Albert Szent-Georgi was never able to cure scurvy with isolated ascorbic acid. In contrast, eating an orange provides whole vitamin C with all the necessary cofactors for optimum absorption.

It is this very concept that lies at the center of the CBD oil from hemp vs. CBD oil from cannabis debate.

While it may be cheaper and more cost-effective to extract CBD from industrial hemp, users may ultimately experience fewer benefits due to the absence of clinically significant levels of terpenes and other compounds which occur in abundance in high-CBD cannabis.

Agricultural hemp is much closer to the kind of cannabis that one would find growing naturally, whereas high-CBD cannabis is hybridized and altered by growers to produce the highest levels of the desired compounds.

Unfortunately, there are no hard facts about the validity of the entourage effect. It is up to each individual to research, consult with medical professionals, and decide for themselves the best path forward.

9.) CBD and THC Have Different Benefits for Pain

Research suggests CBD may be better for inflammation and neuropathic pain, while THC may excel with spasticity and cramp-related pain.

High doses of THC can exacerbate current pain symptoms making micro-dosing with THC a more reasonable pain management strategy.

Many people experience difficulty managing the side effects of THC, and because CBD can mitigate these side effects, some experts to suggest a combination of THC and CBD as a more manageable approach to treating pain.

THC is illegal and carries considerable immediate and long-term cognitive side effects. These include impaired thinking and reasoning, a reduced ability to plan and organize, altered decision-making, and reduced control over impulses.

In addition, chronic use of THC correlates with significant abnormalities in the heart and brain. CBD lacks many of these harmful effects. Given the increasing popularity of medical marijuana, breeders are currently creating strains with higher CBD to THC ratios to minimize these psychoactive side effects.

Overall, the lower health risks of CBD, combined with its efficacy, make it a better candidate for natural supplementation than THC.

10.) CBD Oil Helps Children with Seizures and Epilepsy

Perhaps one of the most exciting applications of CBD oil is its potential impact for adults and children with epilepsy. Individuals who were experiencing dozens of seizures daily have found that CBD can dramatically decrease these numbers.

Considering the shocking increase in children receiving prescriptions for various ailments, CBD oil may provide a non-toxic more natural alternative to pharmaceutical treatments, preventing children from experiencing long term damage or side effects.

CONCLUSION

TAKE AWAY

CBD oil is all the rage right now as a supplement and treatment option.

While the craze around this cannabinoid caught on in the last couple of years, CBD benefits and use date as far back as 2737 B.C. when the Sheng Nung, Emperor of China used it to treat several ailments such as gout and arthritis.

In a very short time, CBD oil has grown rapidly to become a $270 million market, which is expected to be valued at close to $20 billion by 2024. The products range is expanding, and more and more playersgrowers, producers, distributors, and dispensers are also entering the fray.

What is CBD oil? It's the most abundant cannabinoid in the hemp plant. It is also the second most common of 104 cannabinoids found in cannabis plants; only second to THC which produces the feeling of high when you smoke or ingest marijuana.

CBD oil isn't a psychoactive compound, which means that it doesn't have any euphoric effects on the brain. However, it acts by influencing cannabinoid receptors called CB2, which trigger an increase of happy-making hormone, serotonin. With that in mind, CBD oil delivers great health benefits that have been studied extensively.

CBD oil can help with depression and anxiety. It shows anti-anxiety and antidepressant properties thanks to its ability to increase the level of serotonin. This also delivers other benefits like sleep improvement, better mood, reduction of bipolar disorder systems, and much more.

CBD can also help with pain associated with a broad range of ailments, including rheumatoid arthritis, spinal cord injury, Multiple Sclerosis, cancer, chemotherapy, muscle spasms, and depression. When it comes to behavioral conditions, CBD oil can help people beat obesity, lose weight, quit smoking, and rise above anorexia.

In addition, CBD has the ability to interact with the endocannabinoid system (ECS), which makes it the perfect candidate for treating several neurological disorders. These include epilepsies, Alzheimer's disease, Parkinson's disease, ALS, Huntington's disease, PTSD, bipolar disorder and Multiple Sclerosis.

Antioxidant and anti-inflammatory properties of CBD give your body an edge against leukemia, several cancers, acne, Crohn's disease, heart disease, lupus, and much more.

CBD can also lead to physical changes that can help curb glaucoma and other related conditions.Inasmuch as CBD products deliver these incredible benefits, they also comes with a few side effects, including nausea, fatigue, irritability, appetite issues, diarrhea, and tiredness.

CBD is typically extracted in the form of oil, concentrate or powder depending on the producer.

However, it is sold in the form of capsules/pills, tinctures, vape cartridges, or topicals like lotions, balms, and creams. The dosage depends on the concentration of the product, your weigh and desired effects.

Ultimately, the most burning questions would be if CBD oil is actually legal. While it's available pretty in every state, online and in brick-and-mortar stores, the legality of CBD is still fuzzy.